MAXIMUM MUSCULAR FITNESS:

How to Develop Strength Without Equipment

by
Daniel P. Riley
Head Strength Coach
Washington Redskins

Leisure Press
P.O. Box 3
West Point, N.Y.

D1603539

A publication of Leisure Press.

P.O. Box 3, West Point, N.Y. 10996

Copyright© 1982 by Daniel Patrick Riley

All rights reserved. Printed in U.S.A.

ISBN 0-88011-013-9

Library of Congress Number: 81-85634

CONTENTS

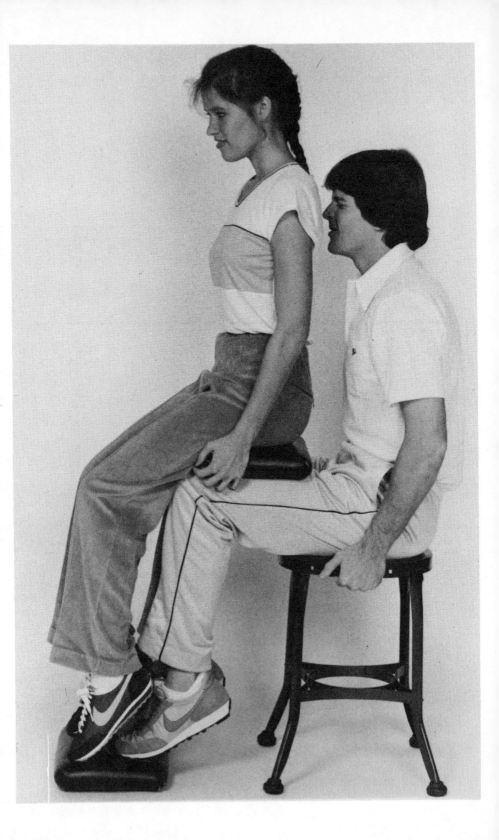

1

WHY MANUAL RESISTANCE?

The methods and techniques for developing muscular fitness have come a long way since the days of Milo of Crotona. Milo was an athlete from ancient Greece. He strengthened his muscles for athletic competition by hoisting a bull upon his shoulders and exercising with it.

Times have obviously changed. The methods employed and the equipment used have gradually evolved through the years. The number of participants abounds. The personal reasons of these individuals for developing muscular fitness are as varied as there are differences in people.

For hundreds of years, the primary purpose of resistance exercise was to prepare soldiers for battle. Life or death often hinged on the warrior's level of fitness. Many hundreds of years passed and eventually Olympic and Powerlifting organizations were formed to accommodate the needs of competitive weight lifters. During this same period, body building began to generate some interest among both recreational and competitive lifters. Body building organizations were formed to provide an avenue for the competitve body builder. For many years, that's all that weight lifting was about—competitive lifting or body building. Coaches refused to allow their athletes to engage in any strength building exercises. They feared an increase in size or strength would adversely affect performance. By the mid 1960's, however, coaches and athletes began to recognize the value of a properly organized program to develop muscular fitness. Almost everyone appeared to be climbing aboard the strength training bandwagon.

Individuals from all walks of life have begun to discount the myths and innuendos concerning muscular fitness. People are finally recognizing that strength training is a terrific tool for improving the quality of their lives. Higher levels of muscular fitness will reduce the chances that an individual will be injured in any physical activity. It will also reduce to a minimum the nagging, muscular aches and pains frequently attendant to daily living. Muscles are firmed and toned-up. By stretching the muscles, flexibility is increased. Higher levels of muscular fitness will also improve athletic performance. In short, proper strength training is enabling people to feel better, perform better, and look better.

In response to the community-wide demand for information on how to best develop muscular fitness, high school and college physical education programs have also experienced a mushrooming interest in strength training. Formal classes are offered in most programs to instruct students and help them develop the tools and understanding to carry-over this interest into their adult lives. In response to this new found interest in developing muscular fitness, weight training equipment companies began producing an assortment of equipment to meet the needs of a broad spectrum of athletic combatants—from wide shouldered football players to petite gymnasts.

Over a generation has passed since strength training was initially introduced to large masses of people. The interest expressed by coaches and athletes is greater than ever and continues to increase. As a result, adults from all walks of life are being exposed to the numerous benefits of a sound muscular fitness conditioning program. The popularity of strength training

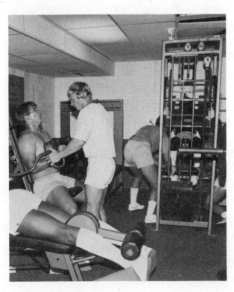

High school and college physical educational programs have also experienced a mushrooming interest in strength training.

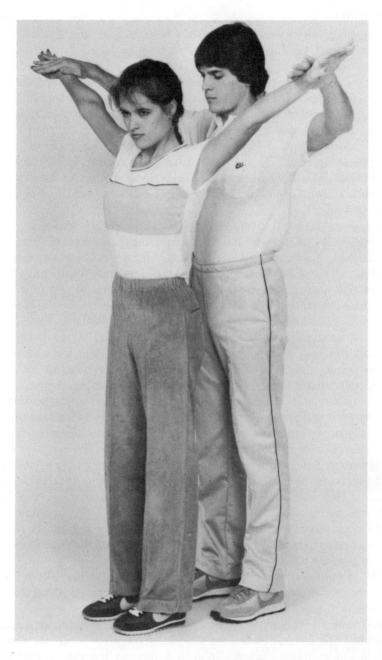

The resistance in MR resistances is provided by a training partner or spotter.

will continue to grow as people see for themselves (and "spread the word") that higher levels of muscular fitness are both desirable *and* attainable.

The interest generated in strength training by all sorts of people has created some distinct problems for everyone. Coaches and athletes frequently find that the facilities available at their schools are inadequate. The strain placed upon the facilities has caused congestion, overcrowding, lack of organization and hardships for the entire program. In-season training is almost impossible and usually nonexistent.

The working man or woman finds it difficult to maintain a regular routine of training. By the same token, it is often inconvenient for housewives to leave their homes and their responsibilities. Another factor is expense. The cost of health clubs often prohibits many people from joining such facilities.

It appears that we've created a problem. There are large masses of people from all walks of life who have developed their own personal interest in conditioning their muscles. Unfortunately, for one reason or another, they are unable to sustain regular participation in a muscular fitness program.

But all is not lost. There is a way out of this dilemma for everyone. I call it manual resistance. It's a form of resistance exercise designed to stimulate maximum gains in muscle strength and endurance. Manual resistance (MR) offers a productive alternative to anyone interested in the benefits of resistance exercise . . . the teacher, the coach, the athlete, the student, the career person, the housewife, etc. MR can serve as a substitute for other, more conventional forms of resistance—bar, dumbbells, machines.

The resistance in MR exercises is provided by a training partner or spotter. Anyone who knows how to spot the exercises can overload the muscles and help strengthen them in the same manner that the other more conventional forms of resistance can.

Remember that two things are needed to strengthen a muscle: *resistance* and *overload*. The muscle is *overloaded* if it is forced to work harder each workout with more *resistance* or reps. The type of resistance is not the key. The muscles do not know if you're using a sandbag, rocks, or a dumbbell.

There are structural differences between and among all of the various types of equipment available. Regardless of the type of equipment used, the key to progress is how you use the equipment.

MR can provide the same overload that a dumbbell or barbell can. Don't view the resistance being supplied by a training partner as anything different from that of any traditional form of resistance.

If a variety of equipment is available, MR can be used to supplement a workout. MR can add variety to a workout and significantly increase the number of exercises available. In fact, some exercises can be performed more effectively using MR, regardless of the equipment available.

8

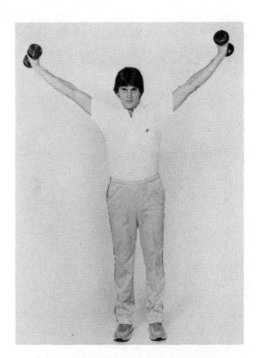

Conventional forms of resistance offer nothing more than manual resistance (MR) can provide.

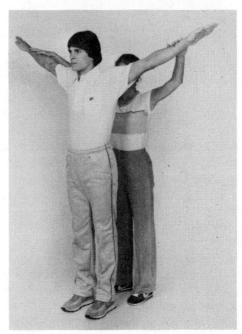

Your muscles don't know if you're using a sandbag, rocks, a machine, or a dumbbell.

WHAT ARE THE MAJOR ADVANTAGES OF USING MR?

There are many advantages to using MR. Some of the more obvious reasons include:

* No equipment is required to perform the exercises.
* Large numbers of individuals can be trained simultaneously.
* The muscles can be worked maximally each rep.
* The speed of the exercise can be controlled.

Since no equipment is needed, these exercises can be performed any time and any place. A coach, for example, can administer the program on the field, court or diamond, or at the end of a practice. A physical education instructor can hold his class indoors or outdoors. The career person can perform the exercises during lunch hour. The housewife can wait until all the kids are asleep and exercise right at home. The point to be remembered is that MR exercises can be performed at any time and any place. Waiting to use equipment is no longer a problem with MR.

Two people or two hundred people can perform the exercises simultaneously. One person exercises while the other supplies the work load. To the coach or the P.E. instructor who has experienced the frustration of overcrowded facilities, MR is a god-send. Due to congestion, for example, most students only have the time to perform a few exercises in a 45 minute weight training class. This is not a problem with MR. In a 30 minute time period, two people can easily spot and perform at least 13 exercises.

Once an individual has been exposed to MR, conditioning the muscles can be a lifelong activity. No longer will a lack of equipment be an obstacle. Maximum resistance can be obtained during the raising and lowering phase of each rep. If the lifter can raise 80 pounds on the first rep, the spotter can apply 80 pounds worth of resistance. If the lifter can only lift five pounds of resistance on the last rep, the spotter can accommodate this decreasing strength level accordingly.

Why is this an advantage? Because it reduces the level of strength closer to the point of zero. More of the muscle is brought into play, thereby causing a greater overload.

The speed of the MR exercise can be controlled. The rate of resistance during the raising phase will be dictated by the amount of resistance applied by the spotter. The lifter's partner or the instructor can decide upon the speed of exercise during the raising phase.

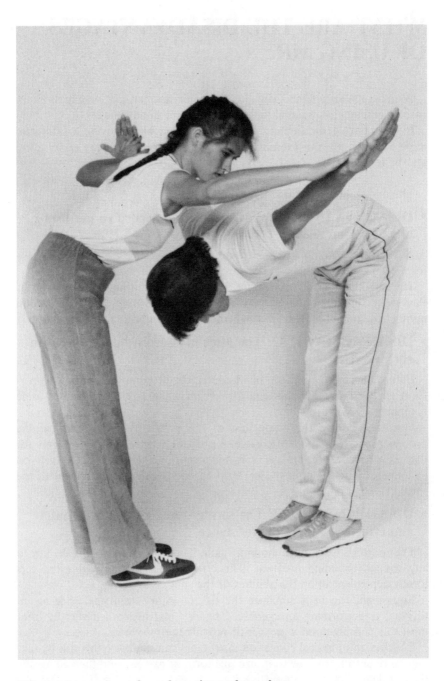

MR exercises can be performed any time and any place.

WHAT ARE THE DISADVANTAGES OF USING MR?

With all its advantages, MR also has some distinct disadvantages. Every type of equipment available has advantages and disadvantages.

By recognizing the limitations of MR, it can help provide a safer and more effective form of exercise. A better understanding of the exercise will also be realized.

The major limitations of MR include:

- **DISADVANTAGE #1: Two people are needed to perform any MR exercise.**

A lifter and a training partner to apply the resistance are required to perform each exercise. This can be a problem for some fitness enthusiasts.

The working person may want to work out during the lunch hour. Perhaps a training partner is unavailable. Possibly a fitness class has an odd number of students. This will leave one student without a training partner.

- **DISADVANTAGE #2: The lifter must learn how to perform each exercise.**

Before maximum gains can be obtained, the lifter must learn how to perform each exercise. This is also a problem when any new exercise (using equipment) is performed.

However, due to the uniqueness of this style of exercise, the learning process of performing a MR exercise probably creates more problems for the inexperienced lifter than will a conventional exercise performed on equipment. The lifter must also learn to coordinate the exercise with the spotter.

- **DISADVANTAGE #3: The spotter must learn how to safely and effectively apply the resistance.**

The spotter's job is even more difficult. The training partner is the key to any strength building program. The effectiveness of any MR exercise is totally dependent upon the abilities of the spotter.

Equipment can help minimize the risk of injury occurring while an individual is performing an exercise. The risk increases whenever the lifter must rely entirely upon a partner to provide the resistance.

Coaches and physical education instructors can minimize this risk by taking the time to learn how to utilize this form of exercise and then educating their athletes and students sufficiently.

It's just like teaching a student-athlete how to block, tackle, perform back somersaults, and do other potentially dangerous skills. Everything demands proper instruction. The instructor should initially treat MR exercise as any other potentially dangerous activity.

Remember, it is the ability of the spotter that dictates the quality of the exercise. There is a specific skill that is required. Some spotters develop a high skill level to spot effectively, while some develop lower skill levels.

An educated lifter will immediately notice the skill level of the spotter. A lower skill level will obviously decrease the effectiveness of the exercise. The spotter must pay strict attention to "responsibilities of the spotter" provided on pages 21-25.

• DISADVANTAGE #4: The lifter may be significantly stronger than the spotter.

After pairing off your students, it's possible that one training partner may be significantly stronger than the other. This can present a problem for the weaker individual.

The spotter has four alternatives while applying resistance to a lifter who is significantly stronger (than the spotter).

- If it is an exercise performed with the upper body, additional resistance can be held by the lifter. Books, paperweights, and so on can be held in the lifter's hands to make the spotter's job easier.
- The lifter can be required to allow more time for the raising phase of the exercise. Allow 2-4 seconds for the raising phase instead of 1-2 seconds.
- De-emphasize the lowering phase until the lifter has reached an adequate fatigue level. Allow 2 seconds to lower the resistance instead of 4 seconds.
- Perform the exercise one leg or one arm at a time.

DISADVANTAGE #5: Accountability

The lifter may ask, "How will I know how much strength I'm gaining from workout to workout?" Unfortunately, accountability will always be a problem. With MR, you cannot record and evaluate strength gains as you can with a barbell or plate-loading machine. You are forced to rely upon your spotters to do their job. When they do, the lifter will be assured of gaining strength.

Point: Sure, there are limitations to manual resistance. We believe, however, that these limitations can be overcome by instructors who are willing to invest a little time in developing the ability to teach these exercises and in providing as much supervision as possible during their execution.

Unfortunately, many instructors have neither the time nor the interest to prepare themselves to handle this area of conditioning. In some programs, the kids know more about strengthening the muscles than the instructors.

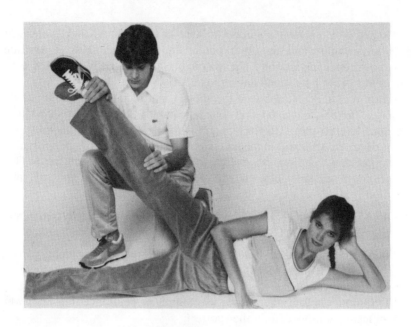

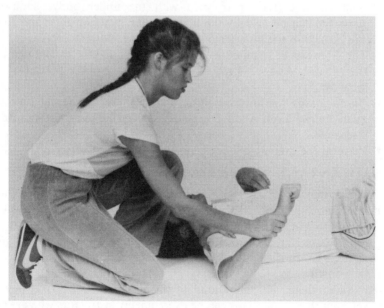

The effectiveness of any MR exercise is dependent to a great extent upon the abilities of the spotter.

Because of the risk involved, coaches and teachers should not expose their athletes and students to this style of training unless they are willing to assume the following responsibilities.

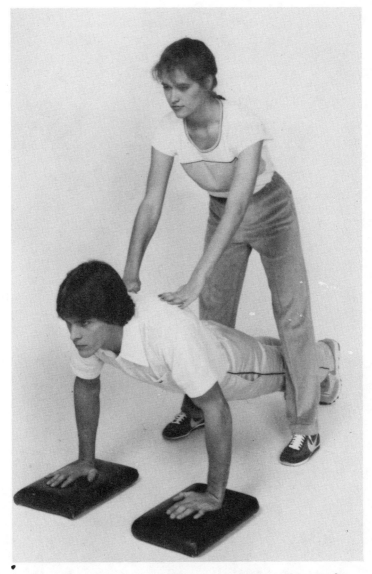

Strict adherence to the MR guidelines is essential for positive results.

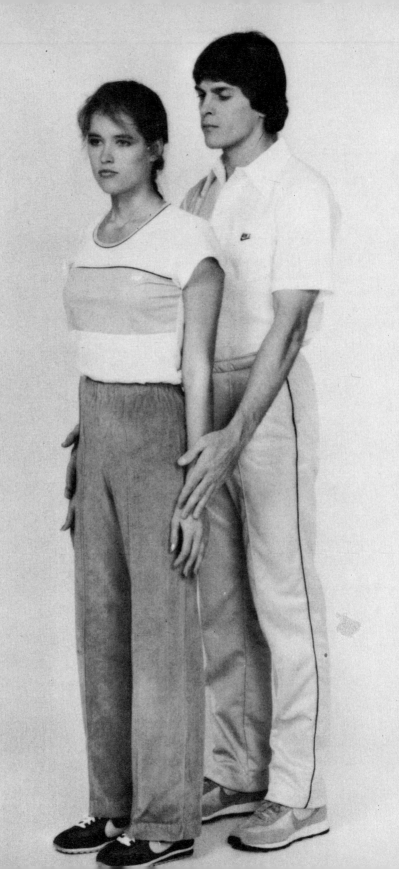

2

GUIDELINES FOR PERFORMING AND TEACHING MANUAL RESISTANCE EXERCISES

HOW TO PERFORM MR EXERCISE

While performing MR exercise, the following guidelines should be used to perform each exercise.
- Perform 12 repetitions or continue exercising for approximately 40 to 70 seconds.
- Perform only one set of each exercise.
- Take four seconds for the lowering phase.
- Allow from one to two seconds to execute the raising phase of each exercise. This phase will include moving from the starting position and pausing in the contracted position momentarily.
- Exercise 2-3 times a week while alternating days.
- Change the order regularly. The order is not important.

WHO SHOULD DO WHAT? THE LIFTER'S RESPONSIBILITIES

For manual resistance to be safe and effective, the lifter must assume some responsibilities during the execution of each repetition. These responsibilities include the following four rules:

Rule #1: Communication with the spotter is essential.

Total cooperation and coordination between the lifter and the spotter are essential. For maximum gains and safety, you may have to tell the spotter how to provide more efficient resistance.

Cooperation with the spotter is needed for smooth and even resistance. Until the spotting and lifting skills have been mastered, the lifter may have to talk to the spotter. For example, "You're not giving me enough resistance," or "You're pulling too hard in the stretched positions."

Rule #2: Keep tension on the muscles.

The relief of the tension for just an instant will allow the muscle to momentarily rest—and make the exercise less productive. Allowing the muscles to relax briefly is a common occurrence while performing an exercise similar to the side lateral raise. When the exercise is properly performed, the hands do not touch the sides of the legs in the starting position of each repetition. This exercise is performed incorrectly if the hands are allowed to touch the sides of the legs. When the hands touch the sides of the legs, the shoulder muscles are given a brief rest. This will make the exercise less productive.

Another example would be the conventional push-up exercise. The muscles are allowed a brief rest if the chest, thighs, or mid-section touch the ground. Ideally, the hands should be elevated off the ground to prevent resting between repetitions.

Rule #3: Pause momentarily in the contracted position.

The lifter should hold the contracted position momentarily during the execution of each repetition. If the lifter doesn't hold this position momentarily, she/he will not maximally develop the muscle at each point during that range of motion.

Also because the lifter can lower more resistance than she/he can raise, she/he must give the spotter ample time to begin applying more resistance during the transition from the raising phase of the exercise to the lowering phase. An example of this concept is the bent over side lateral raise. The

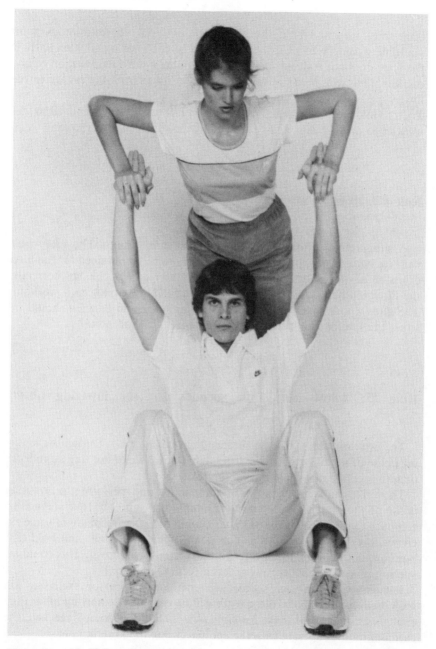

If you do not hold the contracted position, you won't exercise the muscle maximally through its full range of motion.

lifter must stop and hold the contracted position momentarily. A good guideline would be to hold the contracted position for a count of 1001. If the lifter does not concentrate on pausing in the contracted position of any exercise, there will be a bouncing effect or a recoil from the raising to the lowering phase.

Point: Hold any contracted position for a count of 1001 and allow the muscles to develop maximally throughout their full range of motion.

Rule #4: Exert an all-out effort.

A submaximal effort will produce submaximal results. The lifter must work as hard as possible if maximum gains are to be obtained. If the lifter exerts an all-out effort and the training partner applies the MR correctly, the lifter will be assured of maintaining or gaining strength each workout. The lifter who is not interested in obtaining maximum benefits should instruct the spotter to apply the MR at a desired level of intensity.

Rule #5: Allow *only* four seconds for the lowering phase.

The lifter can lower more resistance than he can raise. During the lowering phase of some exercises, the lifter may be capable of exerting more force than the spotter can apply during the first few reps.

The lifter must cooperate with the spotter and perform the lowering phase of the exercise evenly and smoothly, allowing only four seconds to complete this portion of the exercise. During the lowering phase of some exercises, the lifter could stop at any point, if he so desired, and hold that position, not allowing the spotter to pull or push him down. This could invite injury and make the exercise less effective.

Remember that in each succeeding repetition, the person exercising will grow weaker. Eventually the spotter will be capable of applying more than enough resistance during the lowering phase. Until this point is reached, the exerciser must cooperate with the spotter during the lowering phase.

THE SPOTTER'S RESPONSIBILITIES

It should be more than obvious to anyone interested in MR of the value of a properly educated training partner. The effectiveness of MR exercise is almost totally dependent on the abilities of the spotter.

It cannot be emphasized enough how important it is for the instructor to thoroughly educate the participants. For the exercise to be safe and effective, the spotter should strictly adhere to the guidelines outlined herein. The major responsibilities of the spotter include the following:

Rule #1: Communication whenever necessary and constant coordination with the lifter.

Pay attention to the execution of every repetition. The lifter's safety is the spotter's primary concern. How the spotter applies the MR dictates the quality and safety of each exercise.

The spotter should make corrections if needed and provide verbal encouragement for motivation. If the lifter is not strictly adhering to the exact methods prescribed, the spotter should correct the lifter immediately.

Rule #2: *Do not* apply maximum resistance during the first few reps.

The first few reps of each exercise should be used to warm up the muscles involved. This will also help to begin gradually fatiguing the muscles involved so that when the lifter does exert an all-out effort, the muscle will be adequately fatigued. This will decrease the potential for injury.

Point: If maximum resistance is applied on the first few reps, injury could result. Less than maximum resistance is required on the first few reps.

Rule #3: Vary the resistance of each rep during the raising phase.

Once the muscles are warmed up, the spotter should learn to apply as much resistance as the lifter can safely and effectively handle at each point during the raising phase. All movements should be smooth and controlled. This is the most difficult aspect of manual resistance to master.

The amount of resistance that a lifter needs during the raising phase of one rep will actually vary. The bones and muscles are a system of levers. The changing positions of the bones and muscles create leverage advantages and disadvantages. These advantages and disadvantages will require more or less resistance by the spotter.

An example of the leverage system is the conventional push-up exercise. The lifter requires more resistance as the arms straighten. He requires less resistance as the arms bend. Another example of the leverage system can be observed while spotting the side lateral raise. It's obvious that the lifter gradually grows weaker (requires less resistance) as the arms are raised away from the body and weakest in the contracted position.

The spotter should learn to gradually increase or decrease the resistance accordingly to accommodate these changing "strength curves." If the resistance is being applied correctly, the resistance should feel constant to the lifter. The lifter is adding exactly as much resistance as the spotter can raise at each point during the raising phase. If too much resistance is applied at any point, the lifter will be unable to move momentarily. He will be forced to stop the exercise, jerk, or use cheating movements to continue the exercise. If not enough resistance is applied, the exercise will be less productive than it could be.

The spotter should also be aware that the lifter is gradually fatiguing with each succeeding repetition. If the resistance is properly applied, the amount of resistance will decrease with each rep. If the spotter applies the resistance correctly, she/he may only have to apply a few pounds of resistance on the last rep or two. On some exercises, the lifter may be unable to even raise the weight of his arms.

Point: It is the spotter's job to apply just the right amount of resistance at each point during the raising phase.

Rule #4: Smooth transition from the raising phase to the lowering phase.

The person applying the resistance should adjust the amount of resistance at the point of transition from the raising phase to the lowering phase. It should be realized that the lifter can lower more than she/he can raise. That's why it's important for the lifter to pause momentarily in the contracted position. This gives the spotter ample opportunity to begin smoothly applying the additional work load for the lowering phase.

Spotters can't make a sudden change from the raising to the lowering phase or the lifter will be unable to hold the contracted position momentarily. She/he won't make a smooth transition. There would be a sudden drop which wouldn't allow the muscle to be exercised maximally at each point. It may also invite possible injury.

Rule #5: Add more resistance during the lowering phase.

Due primarily to gravity, the lifter can lower more weight than she/he can raise. The spotter should learn to apply more resistance during the lowering phase. If too much resistance is added, the lifter won't be able to resist in the down phase for four seconds. If too little resistance is applied, the lifter could stop at any point during the lowering phase and hold that position for several seconds.

Because the lifter is so much stronger during the lowering phase, there must be a mutual cooperation between the lifter and spotter. The same leverage advantages and disadvantages that exist during the raising phase of each exercise apply to the lowering phase. The person applying the MR must also remember that the lifter is gradually fatiguing each rep.

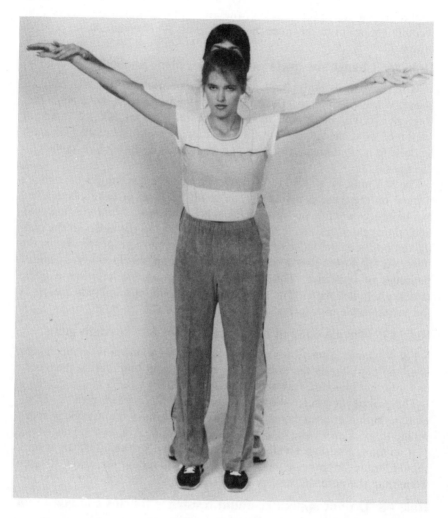

Spotters should make a smooth transition from the raising phase to the lowering phase.

The spotter should learn to apply as much resistance as the lifter can resist while allowing four seconds to lower the weight. If too much resistance is applied during the lowering phase, the lifter would be unable to allow four seconds to perform the lowering movement. This could invite possible injury.

Rule #6: Change the angle of resistance being applied.

Most movements in the body are rotary in nature. Most muscles contract about an axis of rotation. They pull on the bones to form movements that form an arc. For the muscle to be most effectively exercised, the angle of resistance must change through the execution of each repetition. This must be done to accommodate the changing angle that the muscle(s) is pulling on the bone.

The MR must be applied to coincide with the changing angles of each arc formed by the muscles involved. The changing angle of resistance applied can be observed while performing the side lateral raise. In the starting position, the angle of resistance must be perpendicular to the body. In the contracted position, the angle of resistance will be almost perpendicular to the floor. As the lifter raises his/her arms, the spotter should gradually adjust the angle of resistance. This concept will apply almost any time a single muscle group is isolated. The spotter should develop the ability to recognize the correct angle of resistance.

Rule #7: Provide enough resistance to stimulate strength gains.

For maximum gains, the spotter needs to apply as much resistance as the lifter can exert during the execution of each exercise, both during the raising and lowering phase of each repetition.

The goal of the lifter will dictate how intense the exercise must be. Many exercise enthusiasts neither need nor desire optimum results. They aren't willing to exert an all-out effort and don't need to.

If anything less than an all-out effort is exerted by the lifter, the spotter should insure to provide enough resistance to allow the lifter to gain strength at the pace she/he desires.

Rule #8: Do not apply maximum resistance for any exercise in an all-out manner during the first few workouts.

Gradually increase the intensity of exercise in each succeeding workout until the techniques required for each exercise have been mastered.

Rule #9: When necessary, apply less resistance as the lifter approaches the muscle's stretched position.

While performing some exercises, the spotter should learn to gradually decrease the amount of MR being applied as the lifter approaches and eventually reaches the muscle's stretched position. Injury could result if too much resistance is applied in the stretched position of the muscles being exercised.

The spotter should sacrifice the application of maximum resistance to gain maximum stretching and prevent injury. A good example is the neck flexion exercise. The lifter will not relax and stretch the neck muscles if too much resistance is applied. To get the lifter into a relaxed and stretched position (safely), the spotter should begin to gradually decrease the amount of manual resistance as the lifter approaches the neck stretched position. It should be a smooth and gradual transition.

The spotter is applying too much resistance near or at the stretched position if the lifter:

- doesn't reach a completely relaxed and stretched position at the end of each rep;
- stops short of the stretched position;
- feels the need to pull back in the stretched position to prevent hyper-stretching.

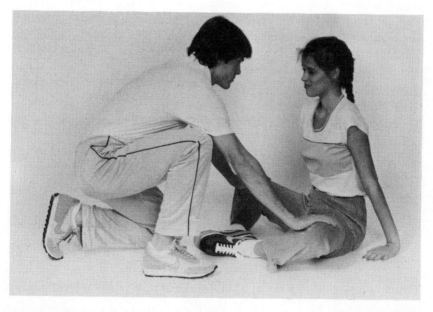

An injury may result if too much resistance is applied in the stretched position of certain exercises.

THE INSTRUCTOR'S RESPONSIBILITIES

Rule #1: Thoroughly read the responsibilities of the spotter and lifter.

The instructor should develop an in-depth understanding of how to apply the MR concepts. These exercises can be spotted and performed in a haphazard manner. Unfortunately, more often than not, this is the rule rather than the exception.

If this occurs the potential results from the exercise will be reduced. Risk of injury to the lifter will be increased.

Point: Thoroughly read the guidelines enclosed and develop a detailed understanding of how to safely and effectively spot and perform each exercise.

Rule #2: Perform the exercises with another instructor in order to develop the skills needed to spot and perform each exercise.

It's obvious to every coach and physical educator that doing something is better than talking about it. Unfortunately, few instructors are willing to actually practice doing the MR exercises. The exact skills to apply the resistance and perform the exercises will not be developed unless the instructor practices what he preaches.

Point: There is nothing overly demanding about the skills needed to spot and perform each exercise. Something will be lost, however, from the instructor to the student if the instructor doesn't experience some of the problems encountered.

Rule #3: If unwilling to perform the exercises, at least practice the spotting procedures until they are mastered.

Every instructor knows that you don't have to demonstrate a back somersault to teach it. If you can't do a back somersault and you are going to teach it, you better make sure you've done your homework.

Nothing compares with a practical background combined with the technical expertise required to perform a skill. The same holds true with MR exercise.

Point: The instructor better be prepared to at least master the skills of the spotter before exposing students to any of this material. The justification is obvious—risk of injury to the lifter and the liability of the instructor.

Rule #4: Minimize the loss in the interpretation of this information from the instructor to the students.

The instructor's first responsibility is to adhere to the aforementioned rules. The eventual quality of MR exercise performed by the participants will be determined by how well the instructor prepares himself/herself and

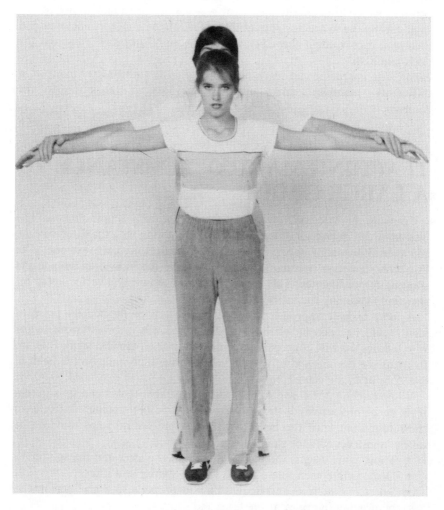

Nothing compares with a practical background combined with the technical expertise required to perform a skill. The same holds true with MR exercise.

by how well that information is taught to the students. This is not the type of information that is posted on the weight room bulletin board. Initially, constant supervision by the instructor is necessary to eliminate any confusion. Ideally the instructor should discuss all of the concepts enclosed and then spot each student through the exercises until they have mastered the skills required.

Point: The instructor can teach one thing and the student may interpret it differently. Instructors must minimize the loss in translation to the students.

TEACHING MANUAL RESISTANCE TO A LARGE GROUP

Teaching the MR concept to one person is a fairly simple process. The instructor can discuss all of the pertinent information with the lifter. She/he can then individually supervise the individual through each exercise. The instructor can then become the lifter and have the individual assume the spotting responsibilities. This is the safest and most effective for initial instruction (assuming the instructor is competent).

A more realistic approach from the instructor's or the coach's point of view would be mass indoctrination. This approach involves an instructor who teaches the MR concept to an entire class or an athletic team. P.E. instructors use this method of teaching most of the time while on the field, in the gym, or in the classroom.

While teaching, MR instructors should remember that it can be a potentially dangerous activity if the instructor is not properly prepared. (Refer to the responsibilities of the instructor.) There are several steps that can be taken to instruct MR for the first time.

- Thoroughly discuss the responsibilities of the lifter and the spotter.
- Demonstrate each rule outlined for the spotter and lifter.
- Select one exercise and discuss how to properly spot and perform it, reinforcing the rules of the lifter and spotter.
- Demonstrate how to incorrectly spot and perform an exercise violating the rules outlined for the lifter and spotter.
- Select 2 volunteers from the group and talk them through an exercise.
- Have the group then perform the same exercise.

The instructor should demand that the group follow his/her exact instructions. With a verbal cadence or a visual demonstration, the participant's speed of exercise can be controlled. For example, while performing the side lateral raise, the instructor's arms can be raised and lowered at the exact speed required from the students.

Constant interaction between the group and instructor is necessary. Corrections can be made at any point during the exercise. Remember that the first few sessions should be spent developing the skills required of the spotter and lifter. Do not encourage or allow any all-out efforts initially. Keep the intensity of the exercise low and gradually increase it each meeting.

After the lifter finishes performing the first exercise, bring the group back together. Reinforce the proper techniques, particularly those not being used by the spotter.

Allow the lifter and spotter to reverse roles and continue the same procedure used to instruct the first group of lifters. Teach only a few exercises at a time.

Review the proper spotting and lifting techniques each class. Constant supervision is required by the instructor until the students have mastered the skills needed.

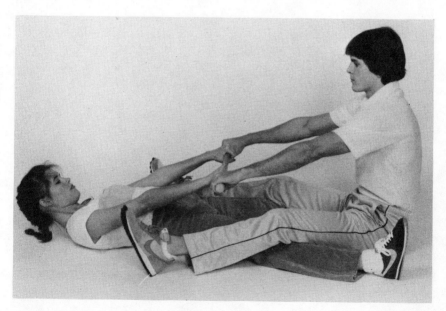

Do not encourage or allow any all-out efforts initially.

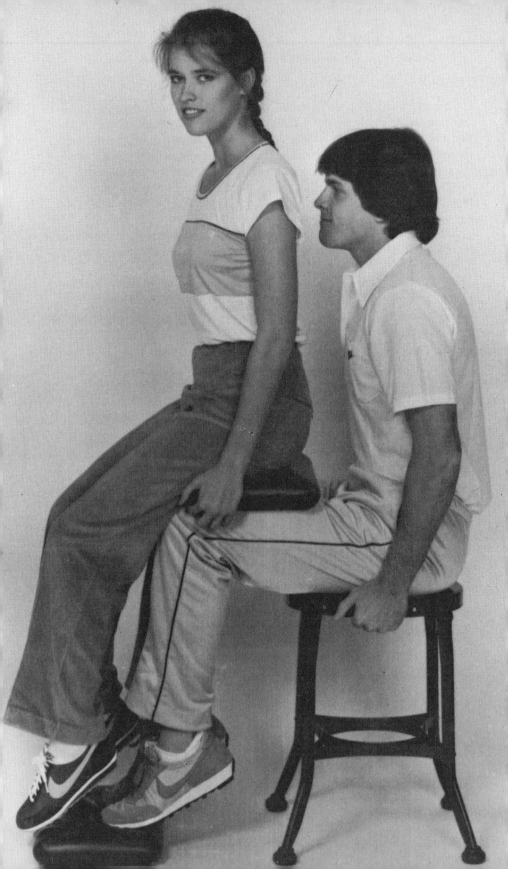

3

MANUAL RESISTANCE EXERCISES

There are a variety of exercises that can be done. There are also some limitations on which ones can be performed effectively. Try to vary the selection of exercises each workout if possible.

The body can be divided into five major segments. They include the lower body, the upper body, the arms, the abdominals and the neck. The manual resistance exercises described in this chapter are categorized by body segments.

LOWER BODY EXERCISES

Hip Abduction

• This is a good exercise to develop the muscles on the outside of the hip and leg.

• In the starting position, the lifter lies on the side with the body extended. The legs should be slightly separated. The upper and lower body remains perfectly aligned throughout the execution of the exercise. Do not allow the upper body to bend forward at the waist.

• The manual resistance can be applied to the side of the leg. If there is a history of knee problems, apply the MR just above the knee.

• During the execution, raise the leg sideward and upward as high as possible and pause momentarily in the contracted position before recovering to the starting position.

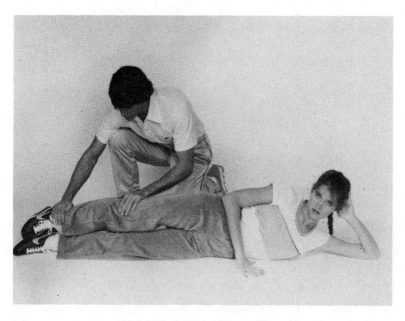

Hip abduction: starting position

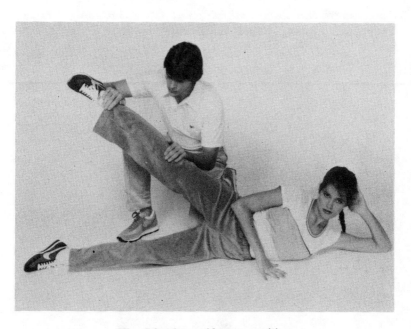

Hip abduction: mid-range position

Hip Adduction

• A good exercise to strengthen the muscles on the inside of the legs. It can also help improve groin flexibility.

• In the starting position, the lifter lies on the back with the legs bent.

• The MR is applied to the inside of the knees. The spotter must use caution as the lifter approaches the stretched position. Injury could result if the spotter applied too much resistance in the stretched position.

• To perform the exercise, raise the knees upward and toward each other to the contracted position. Pause momentarily and return to the starting position.

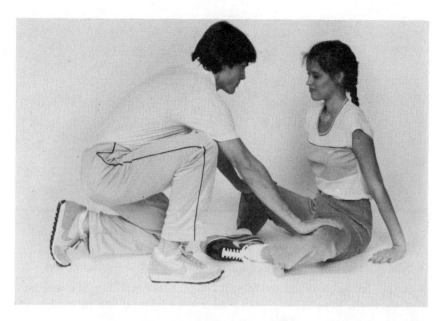

Hip adduction: starting position.

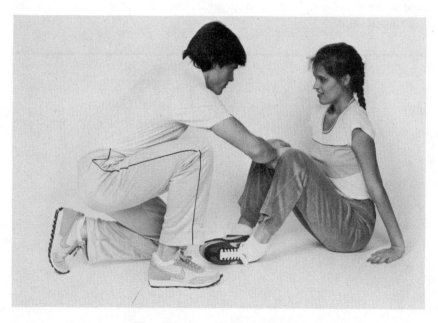

Hip adduction: mid-range position.

35

Hip Flexion

• This is a good exercise to develop the muscles called the hip flexors.

• In the starting position, the lifter is lying on his back. The MR is applied just above the knee. The spotter must move backward and forward as the lifter raises and lowers the leg.

• To perform the exercise flex the hip, raising the knee toward the chest, and pause momentarily in the contracted position before recovering to the starting position.

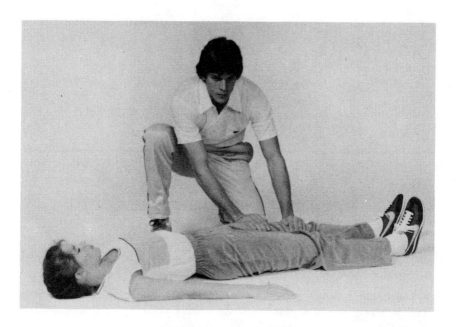

Hip flexion: starting position

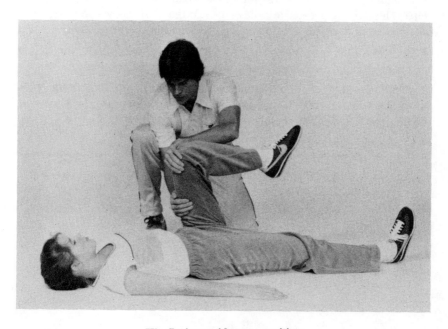

Hip flexion: mid-range position

Squat

• The squat is a general exercise that involves all of the major muscles of the hips and legs. The exercise can be performed one leg at a time. If the exercise is performed with both legs, the spotter is forced to apply the resistance to the hips. The spotter is not strong enough, however, to apply an adequate amount of resistance when both legs are exercised at once.

• The spotter stands on the opposite side of the lifter's leg being exercised. This will help the lifter balance. The person squatting can place an arm around the spotter's shoulder for additional stability.

• Initially, most students do not possess enough strength to perform 12 reps. The training partner may have to help the lifter recover to the starting position until the lifter develops enough strength to perform 12 reps.

• Once the lifter is strong enough to perform 12 reps correctly, the spotter can begin to apply additional resistance to the hips of the lifter.

• While squatting, the lifter should attempt to keep the foot flat and the lower leg perpendicular to the ground. Lower the buttocks to a position behind the feet with the middle of the thigh parallel to the ground.

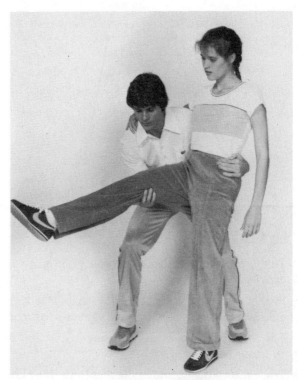

Squat: mid-range position

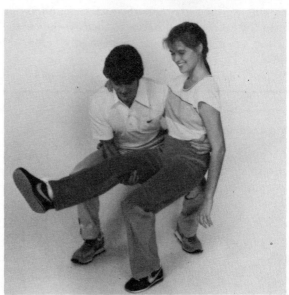

Squat: starting position

Leg Curl

• This is an exercise designed to develop the hamstrings. It is best if each leg is exercised individually.

• In the starting position, the lifter should be lying face down. The toes should be pointed to help increase the range of motion.

• The MR is applied to the backside of the heel or leg. If necessary, use both hands to spot.

• While raising the leg, point the toes toward the knee. Keep the foot in this position until the toes almost touch the ground during the lowering phase. Point the toes at this position to increase the range slightly. Raise the leg as high as possible and pause momentarily before recovering to the starting position.

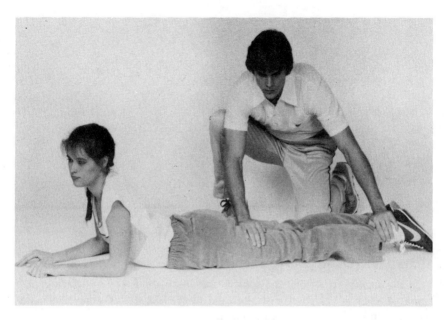

Leg curl: starting position

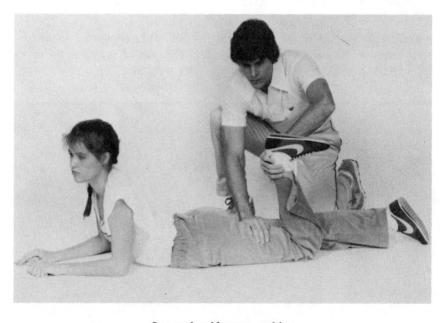

Leg curl: mid-range position

Seated Back Extension

• This a difficult exercise to perform and spot for the lower back muscles.

• In the starting position, the spotter and lifter are seated and facing each other. A stick is held by the spotter and lifter. If a stick is unavailable, interlock hands. The lifter is lying down.

• The spotter should be in a position that allows the lifter to raise and lower the torso. The spotter provides the resistance reciprocally during the raising and lowering phase.

• During the execution, the lifter resists the pull of the spotter while the torso is being pulled away from the floor. The lifter would then pull the torso back to the original position while the spotter resisted.

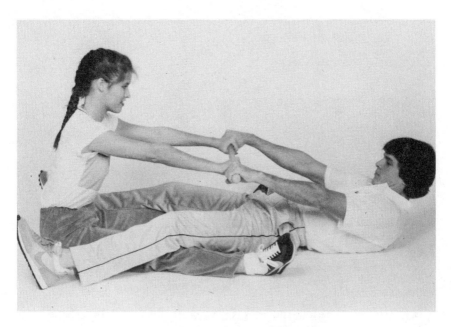

Seated Back Extension: starting position

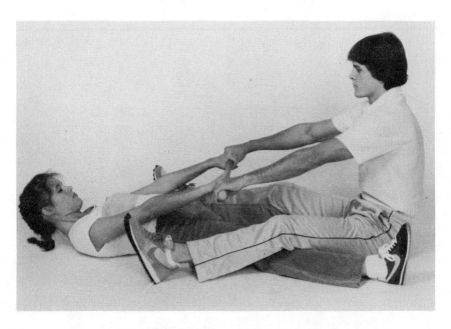

Seated Back Extension: mid-range position

Leg Press

• This is a good exercise to involve the hips and legs. Also difficult to spot and execute correctly.

• In the starting position, the lifter is lying on the back with one foot on the spotter's chest. The arms are extended for balance.

• The training partner's body weight serves as the resistance.

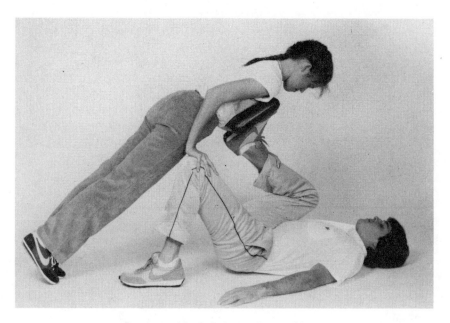

Leg press (single leg): starting position.

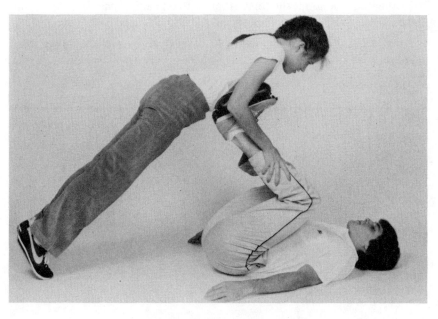

Leg Press (double leg): starting position.

Back Extension

• A good exercise for the lower back muscles. A table or exercise bench is required.

• The lifter's legs and hips must be secured to the table. The body is bent at the waist.

• The MR is applied to the upper back.

• During the execution, the torso is raised to a position parallel to the floor. Pause momentarily and recover to the starting position.

• Extra caution should be used. Most people ignore the lower back muscles. Also, the weight of the lifter's upper body alone may be more than enough weight initially.

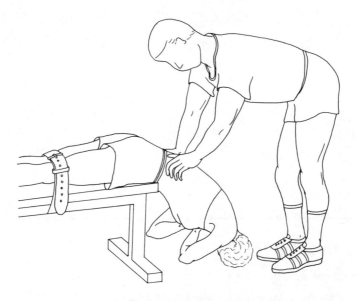

Back extension: starting position.

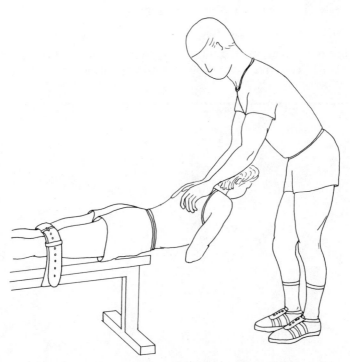

Back extension: mid-range position.

Ankle Rotation In

• An exercise designed to strengthen the inside of the ankle.

• The lifter can be seated or standing. In the starting position, it is best if the heel is slightly elevated off the ground. This allows the foot to rotate more freely. The foot should be rotated outward.

• The MR is applied to the inside of the foot.

• During the execution, the ankle is rotated inward completely and held momentarily before recovering to the starting position.

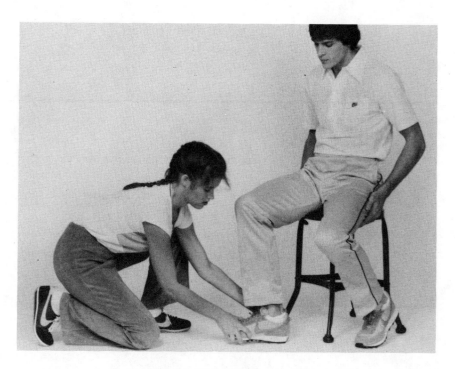

Ankle rotation in: starting position

Ankle Rotation Out

• This exercise is designed to strengthen the muscles on the outside of the leg and ankle.

• The exercise can be performed standing or seated. The foot should be rotated inward in the starting position.

• The MR is applied to the outside of the foot.

• To perform the exercise, rotate the foot outward as far as possible and pause momentarily before recovering to the starting position.

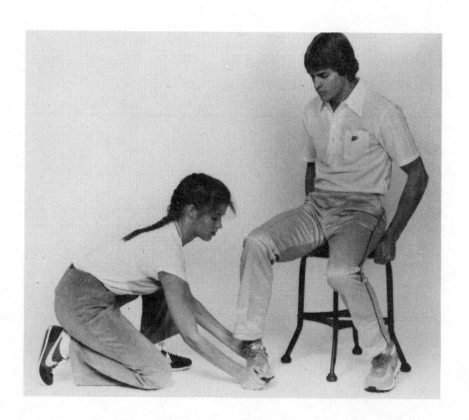

Ankle rotation out: starting position

Ankle Flexion

• This is a good exercise for the muscles on the front side of the ankle and leg.

• In the starting position, the exerciser is seated with the leg extended and the heel elevated slightly. The ankle is relaxed with the toes pointing away from the body.

• The spotter should apply the MR on the top of the foot just below the toes.

• To perform the exercise, flex the ankle completely and pause momentarily before recovering to the starting position.

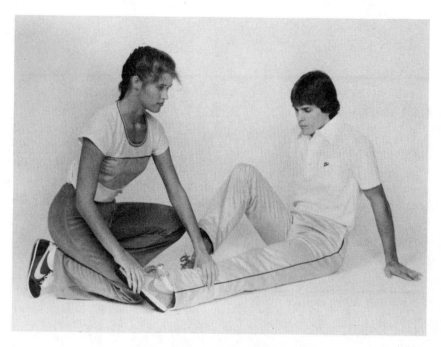

Ankle flexion: starting position

Calf Raises

• This is an exercise designed to develop the calves. It can be performed seated or standing.

• To obtain a stretch in the starting position, the toes must be elevated slightly. The training partner can provide the resistance by sitting on the lifter's lower back or on the knees. The exercise can also be performed one leg at a time (with or without a spotter).

• During the execution, elevate the heel as high as possible and pause momentarily before recovering to the starting position.

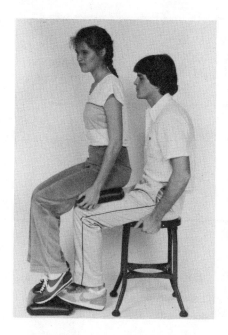

Calf raises (seated): starting position.

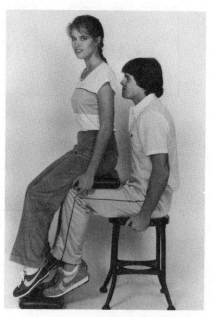

Calf raises (seated): mid-range position.

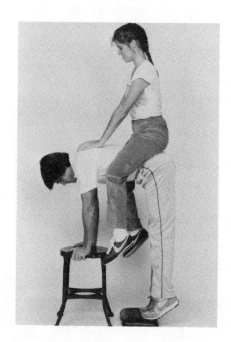

Calf raises (standing): mid-range position.

UPPER BODY EXERCISES

Push-Up

• This is a good exercise for the pushing muscles (chest, shoulders, triceps).

• In the starting position, the lifter should assume a good push-up position. The hands can be elevated to provide maximum stretching and prevent resting in the stretched position.

• During the exercise, the body is lowered to a position where only the chest muscles touch the floor (if pads are unavailable to elevate the hands) and then recover to the starting position. Do not allow the thighs or midsection to touch the floor.

• The MR is applied to the upper back.

• If the lifter is unable to continue the exercise in the conventional push-up position, the modified push-up position can be assumed. If the lifter is unable to perform another repetition correctly, the hands and knees position should be assumed immediately. This will allow the lifter to continue the exercise.

• When the all fours position is assumed, the lifter should move the hands forward of the shoulders. The toes should be elevated. During the lowering phase, the lifter should be leaning forward so that the chest muscles eventually are directly over the hands in the stretched position.

• If the lifter cannot touch the chest to the floor in the all fours position, move the hands forward until the chest can be comfortably lowered to the floor.

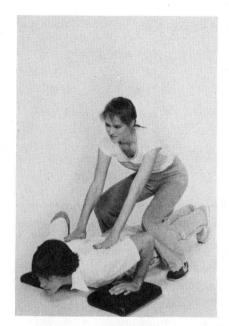

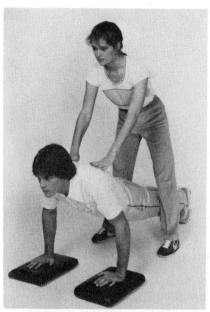

Push-up: starting position

Push-up: mid-range position

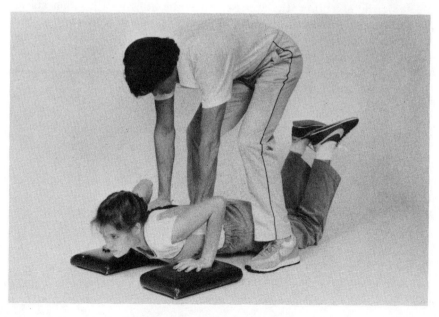

Modified push-up: starting position.

Side Lateral Raise

• This is an exercise for the shoulder muscles.

• In the starting position, the lifter is standing erect with the arms extended and palms facing inward but not touching the sides of the legs.

• The MR is applied to the back of the wrists throughout the execution of the exercise.

• During the execution, the exerciser raises the arms to a position above parallel to the ground and pauses momentarily before recovering to the starting position.

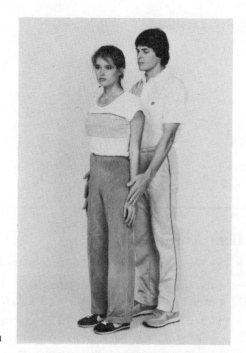

Side lateral raise: starting position

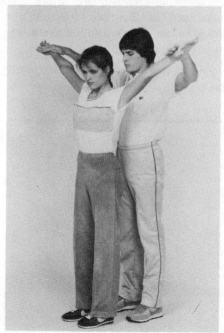

Side lateral raise: mid-range position

Bent Arm Fly

• The bent arm fly is designed to develop the chest muscles.

• In the starting position, the exerciser is lying on the back with the arms bent at 90° and the upper arm perpendicular to the body.

• The MR is applied to the inside of the arm. The exercise is easiest to spot one arm at a time but can be performed with both arms. Because the muscles being exercised are stronger than the muscles used to spot, I'd recommend that less time (2 seconds) be allowed for the lowering phase if both arms are exercised simultaneously.

• To perform the exercise, raise the elbow(s) upward and toward the midline of the body. Pause momentarily and recover to the starting position.

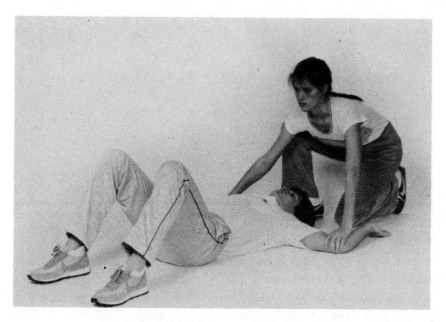

Bent arm fly: starting position

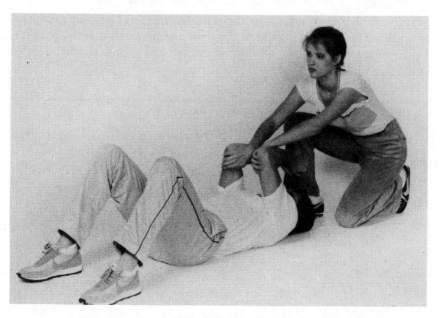

Bent arm fly: mid-range position

Bent Over Side Lateral Raise

• The posterior muscles of the shoulders and upper back are developed while performing this movement.

• In the starting position, the upper body should be bent at the waist and parallel to the ground with the arms extended and hanging downward. The arms are crossed to provide maximum stretching. Do not bend the arms.

• The resistance can be applied to the backside of the wrists or elbows.

• To perform the exercise, raise the arms sideward and upward to a position where the arms are parallel to the floor and perpendicular to the upper body. Pause momentarily in the contracted and return to the starting position.

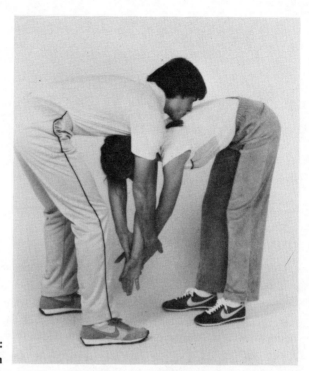

Bent over side lateral raise: starting position

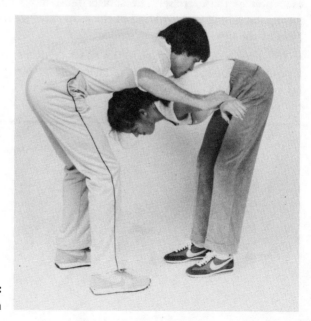

Bent over side lateral raise: mid-range position

Front Raise

- This is another good exercise to develop the muscles of the shoulders.

- In the starting position, the lifter's feet should be staggered for better balance. The body should be erect and remain that way throughout the exercise. The arms are extended and to the rear of the body with the palms facing away. The arms are kept at shoulder width throughout the execution.

- The MR is applied to the *backside* of the *wrists* and hands *throughout* the execution of the exercise. The spotter must move backward and forward during the raising and lowering of the arms. This must be done to allow the arms of the lifter to remain extended.

- To perform the exercise, the lifter raises the arms forward and upward to a position overhead and pauses momentarily before recovering to the starting position.

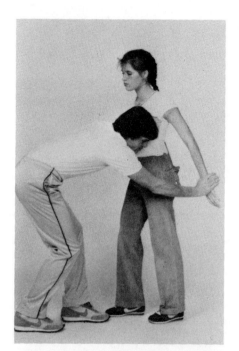

Front raise: starting position

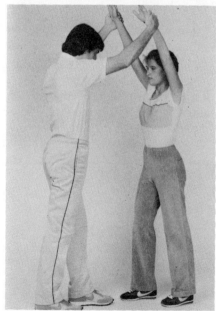

Front raise: mid-range position

Seated Press

• This exercise will primarily develop the shoulder muscles. The chest and triceps muscles are also used.

• In the starting position, the lifter is seated with the legs bent and upper body leaning back slightly. The lean of the upper body will minimize any stress placed upon the lifter's lower back. The spotter must brace the lifter's upper body with a knee.

• The MR is applied to the lifter's hands. The thumbs can be interlocked to form a comfortable grip.

• During the execution, the lifter extends the arms to a position just before locking out and then recovers to the starting position. The forearms should remain perpendicular to the ground throughout the execution of the exercise. If forearms are bent toward the head, the emphasis will be placed on the triceps.

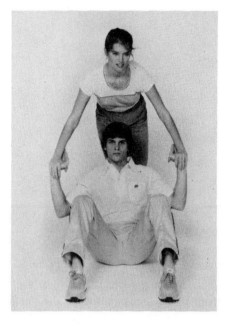 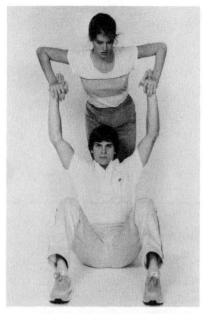

Seated press: starting position   **Seated press: mid-range position**

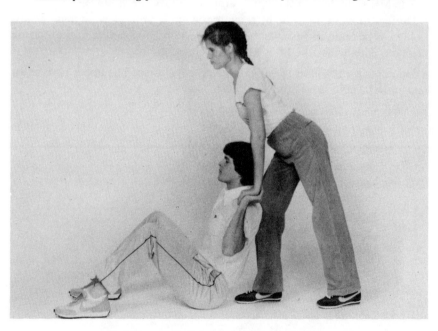

Seated press: lean upper body back slightly.

Bent Over Row

• The bent over row will primarily develop the muscles of the upper back.

• In the starting position, the lifter is bent at the wasit with the right arm bent. The arm is brought across the front of the body to stretch the back muscles in the starting position.

• The MR is applied to the upper arm just above the elbow.

• During the execution, the lifter raises the upper arm sideward and upward as high as possible and pauses momentarily before recovering to the starting position. The higher the lifter raises the elbow the better.

• Do not allow the lifter to extend or rotate the torso. The upper body must remain parallel to the floor.

• Change arms and repeat.

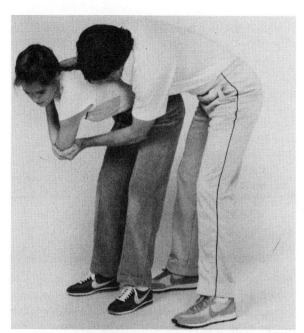

**Bent over row:
starting position**

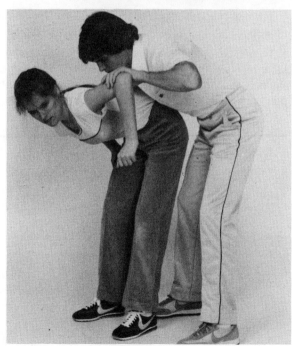

**Bent over row:
mid-range position**

Seated Row

• The seated row will place the emphasis on the upper back and biceps.

• In the starting position, the exercisers should be seated and facing each other. The exercise will be performed simultaneously by both lifters. The participants should be in a position that allows both lifters to pull the stick to the chest and fully extend the arms.

• The resistance is provided reciprocally when one lifter pulls and the other resists.

• To perform the exercise, one lifter pulls the bar to the chest and the other lifter resists while the arms are extended. The roles are then reversed when the person with the arms extended pulls the bar to the chest and the training partner resists while the arms are extended (which completes one rep).

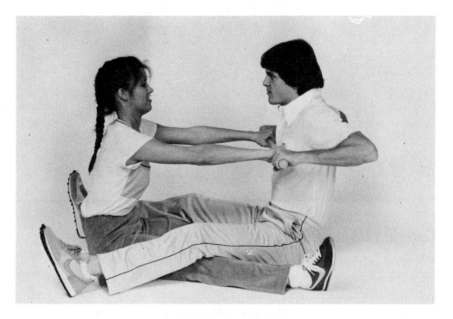

Seated row: starting position

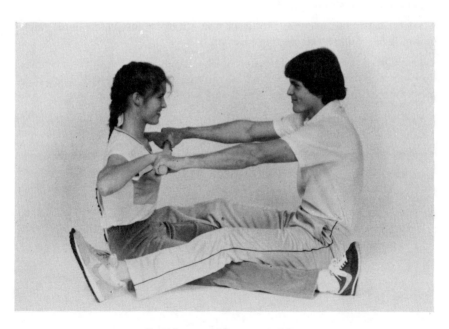

Seated row: mid-range position

External Rotation

• A good exercise for the rotator cuff muscles of the shoulder. Excellent for the pitcher, quarterback, tennis, racquetball or handball, and swimmer.

• In the starting position, the exerciser is lying on the back with the arm bent at 90° and the upper arm perpendicular to the body. The palm of the hand is facing skyward with the arm in a comfortable position. Do not hyperstretch the shoulder.

• To perform the exercise, contract the rotators completely and pause before recovering to the starting position.

• The MR is applied to the palm of the hand throughout the exercise. Caution must be used. A less than maximum effort is suggested. The range of motion of the rotator muscles will vary with the individual.

• Change arms and repeat.

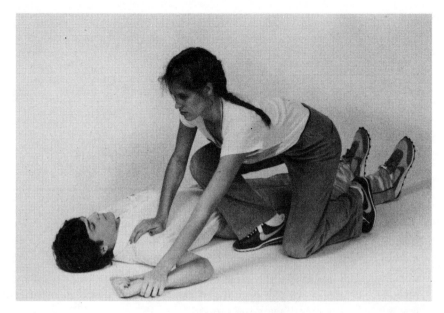

External rotation: starting position

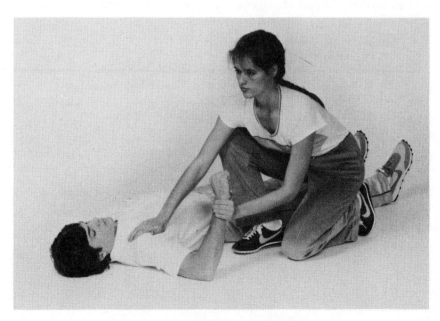

External rotation: mid-range position

Internal Rotation

• Designed to strengthen the backside of the shoulder.

• The starting position is the same position assumed for the external rotation exercise except for the position of the arm. The arm is in a forward position with the palm facing the ground.

• The MR is applied to the back of the hand. Caution must be used. A less than maximum effort is suggested. Range of motion will vary from person to person.

• Change arms and repeat.

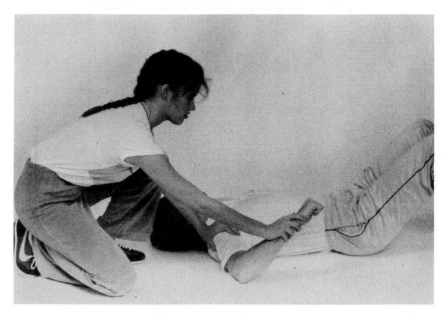

Internal rotation: starting position

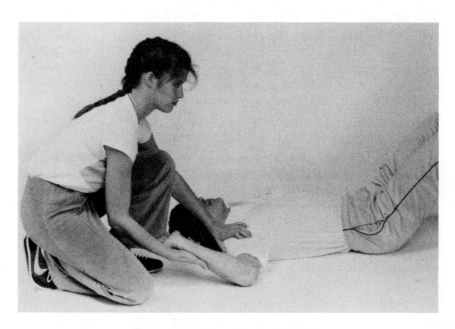

Internal rotation: mid-range position

ARM EXERCISES

Lying Triceps Extension

• This exercise is designed to develop the triceps which are located on the backside of the arm.

• In the starting position, the lifter is lying on the back with the arm bent and the upper arm perpendicular to the ground. The hand is held in a karate chop manner.

• The MR is applied to the side of the hand. The spotter is in a position where the upper leg is resting against the lifter's upper arm. One hand is used to apply the resistance against the side of the lifter's hand while the other holds the lifter's elbow stationary. Do not hyperflex the elbow.

• To perform the exercise, the lifter extends the arm and pauses momentarily before recovering to the starting position.

• The exercise can be performed seated and a towel can be held by the lifter and spotter. The spotter applies the resistance by pulling on the towel.

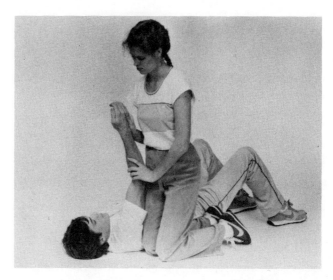

Lying triceps extension: mid-range position

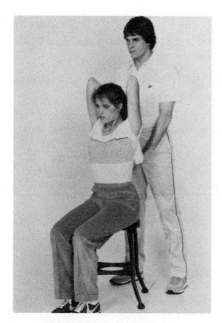

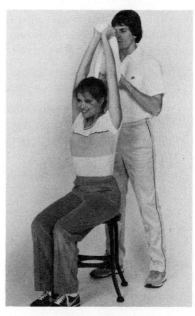

**Seated triceps extension:
starting position.**

**Seated triceps extension:
mid-range position.**

Biceps Curl

• This is a good exercise for the biceps. It is a difficult exercise to spot and perform effectively.

• The starting position is almost identical to the triceps extension. The only difference is the position of the hands. The spotter and lifter must interlock hands to form a comfortable grip.

• The MR is applied to the hand of the lifter. Due to the difficulty in applying enough resistance during the lowering phase, allow less time to lower the resistance and more time for the raising phase.

• To perform the exercise, flex the arm completely and pause before recovering to the starting position.

• The exercise can also be performed with a towel. The spotter is seated and the lifter lying on the stomach with the arm extended. Padding under the elbow may be needed for comfort.

• Change arms and repeat.

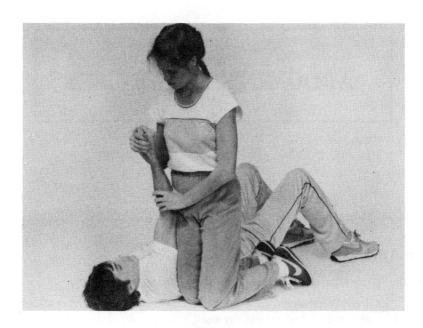

Biceps curl: starting position

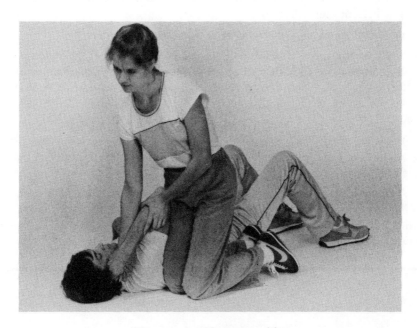

Biceps curl: mid-range position

ABDOMINAL EXERCISES

Sit-Ups

• The sit-up is an excellent exercise for the abdominal muscles.

• In the starting position, tuck the chin and round the upper back. The hands can be interlocked behind the head with the elbows together. The exercise can be made easier by folding the arms across the chest. In the starting position, the lifter must feel tension on the abdominal muscles. The feet can be held or secured.

• The MR can be applied to the front side of the shoulders.

• While performing the exercise, do not take the tension off the abdominals at any time. Raise the body to a desired position and pause momentarily before allowing at least four seconds to recover to the starting position. Keep the upper back rounded at all times to alleviate stress on the lower back.

• There are many variations to the sit-up exercise. A more difficult progression of the sit-up can be performed by using an exercise bench to place the back of the legs upon.

• A twisting sit-up can be performed to involve the rotating muscles of the torso and the oblique muscles on the sides of the abdominal region. The lifter must remain in the twisted position to the right while raising and lowering the torso and then rotate to the left to raise and lower the body.

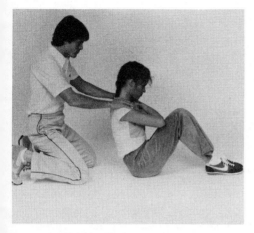

Sit-ups: mid-range position

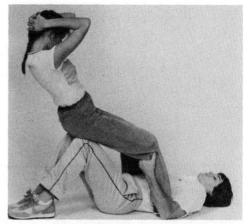

The situps have many variations.

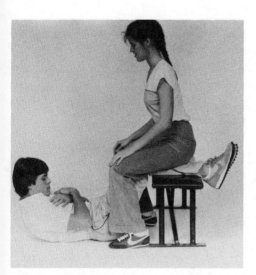

An exercise bench, stool, or chair can be used to make the exercise more difficult.

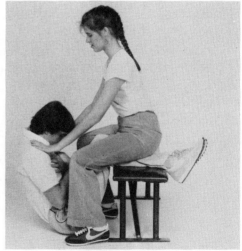

MR can be applied to the front side of the shoulders to make the situp progressively more difficult.

Leg Raise

• Designed to strengthen the abdominal muscles.

• In the starting position, the lifter is on the back with the legs bent and feet not touching the floor. The back is slightly rounded. The hands can grasp something for support.

• If additional resistance is needed, the MR should be applied just above the knees. The spotter must move forward and backward as the lifter raises and lowers the knees.

• To perform the exercise, raise the knees toward the head and pause before recovering to the starting position.

• Do not straighten the legs. This will cause the lifter to arch the back, placing undue stress on the lower back. Keep the legs bent and the back rounded.

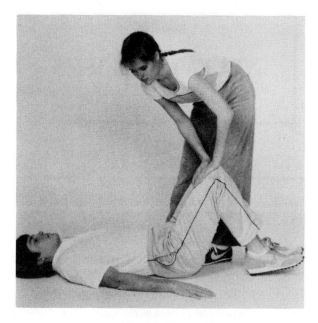

Leg raise: starting position

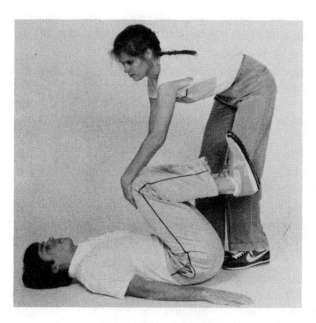

Leg raise: mid-range position

NECK EXERCISES

Lying Neck Flexion

• This is an exercise designed to strengthen the muscles on the front side of the neck. The lifter and spotter must be especially cautious while performing any exercise involving the muscles of the neck. The potential for serious injury exists if the exercise is performed improperly.

• It is easiest to spot when the person performing the exercise is lying on the back. An exercise bench, bleachers, or almost anything can be used to support the lifter.

• In the starting position, the lifter is lying on the bench with the head just off the edge of the bench. The head and neck should be totally relaxed. The spotter is gently applying a mild stretch to the neck flexors.

• The spotter is applying too much resistance in the starting position if the lifter feels the need to pull back or is not completely relaxed. The lifter will not allow the spotter to pull the head into a stretched position if too much resistance is being applied as the lifter approaches and eventually reaches the stretched position. Injury could result if the spotter applies too much resistance and hyperstretches the neck.

• The MR is applied to the forehead. The spotter must take great care to apply the resistance evenly across the forehead.

• During the execution, the lifter must flex the neck until the chin touches the chest and hold this position before recovering to the starting position. Caution must be used as the lifter approaches and eventually reaches the stretched position.

• A less than maximum effort is suggested for any neck exercise. All movements should be performed slower than any other exercise. The slower the better. Allow three repetitions to be performed initially just to warm up the neck muscles. Perform twelve reps thereafter.

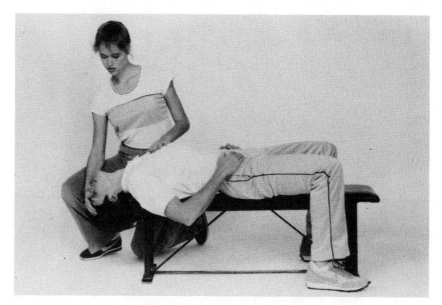

Lying neck flexion: starting position

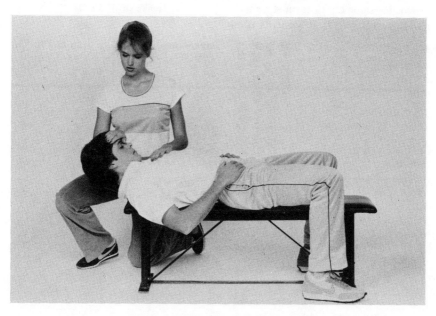

Lying neck flexion: mid-range position

Seated Neck Flexion

• The exercise can also be performed sitting down. This is more difficult to spot and perform than the lying neck flexion.

• All of the same lifting and spotting techniques used for the lying neck flexion also apply when sitting down.

• The lifter is in a more vulnerable position while seated than when lying down. Extreme caution must be used. The lifter flexes only the neck. Do not allow the lifter to pull with the torso.

• The spotter should interlock the fingers and place the hands on the forehead.

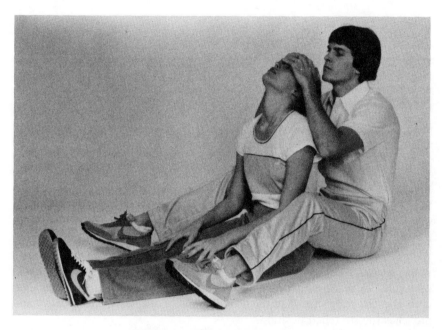

Seated neck flexion: starting position

Neck Extension

• The neck extension exercise is designed to develop the neck extensors, which are located on the back side of the neck and upper back.

• In the starting position, the lifter assumes an all fours position with the chin tucked and neck totally relaxed.

• The MR is applied to the back side of the head. The spotter must be cautious as the lifter approaches and eventually reaches the chin tucked position. The spotter's hand must be in the middle of the lifter's head. Two hands can also be used to spot the exercise.

• The exerciser risks injury at this point and will not relax and stretch the neck muscles if too much resistance is being applied. The training partner must add less resistance than the lifter is capable of resisting as the lifter approaches the stretched position.

• While performing the exercise, the head should be extended as far back as possible and held there momentarily before recovering to the starting position. To assure that the stretched position is reached, the spotter can ask the lifter to relax and roll the head from side to side at the end of each rep.

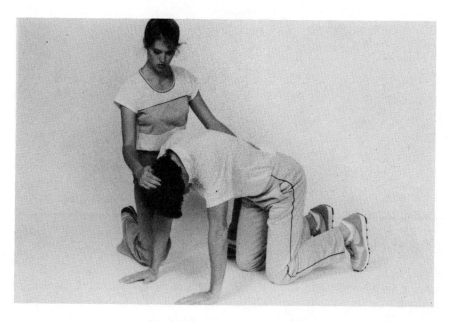

Neck Extension: starting position

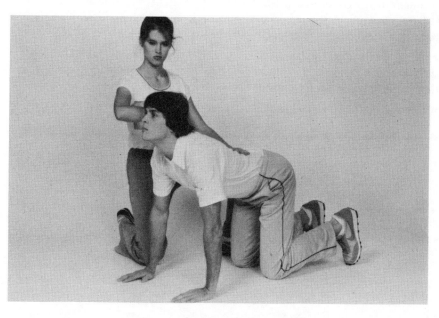

Neck Extension: mid-range position

Lateral Flexion

• This is an exercise to strengthen the side of the neck. It should be performed to the right and the left. We suggest that the resistance be self-imposed to reduce the chance of injury.

• In the starting position, the lifter can be standing or seated. The shoulders should be parallel to the ground and attempt to keep them parallel throughout the execution of the exercise. Looking straight ahead, the head is bent sideward to the left to a comfortable stretched position. The right hand is placed on the right side of the head.

• While performing the lateral flexion (to the right) exercise, move the head sideward to a contracted position and pause momentarily before recovering to the starting stretched position.

• Change sides and repeat the exercise to the left.

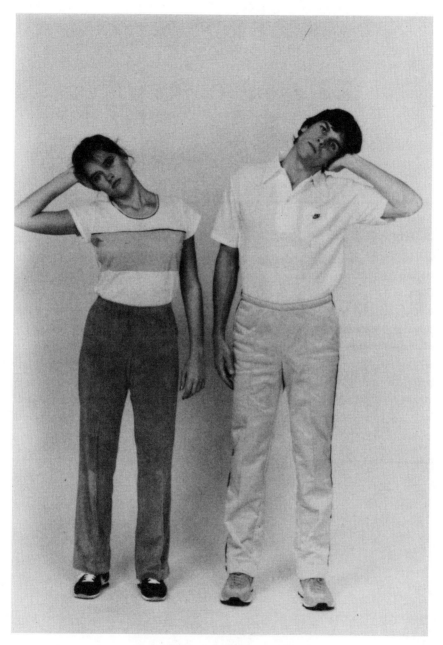

Lateral flexion: mid-range position

Shrugs

• The shoulder shrug is designed to develop the trapezius (traps). It is a strong and powerful muscle located on the back of the neck and upper back.

• The exercise can be best performed if the exerciser is standing with the arms extended and holding a stick. An over and under grip can be used. If a stick is unavailable, the hands can be interlocked.

• The resistance is applied with the body weight of the training partner. A problem that exists is the spotter's body weight may not be enough. If it is too much, the spotter's legs can be bent to make it easier for the lifter.

• To perform the exercise, shrug the shoulders as high as possible and pause before recovering to the starting position.

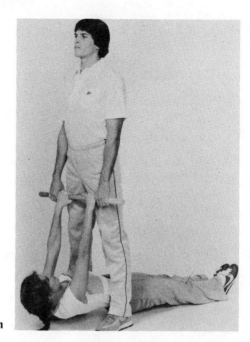

Shrugs: starting position

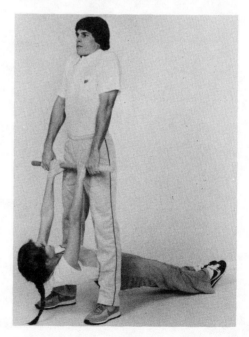

Shrugs: mid-range position

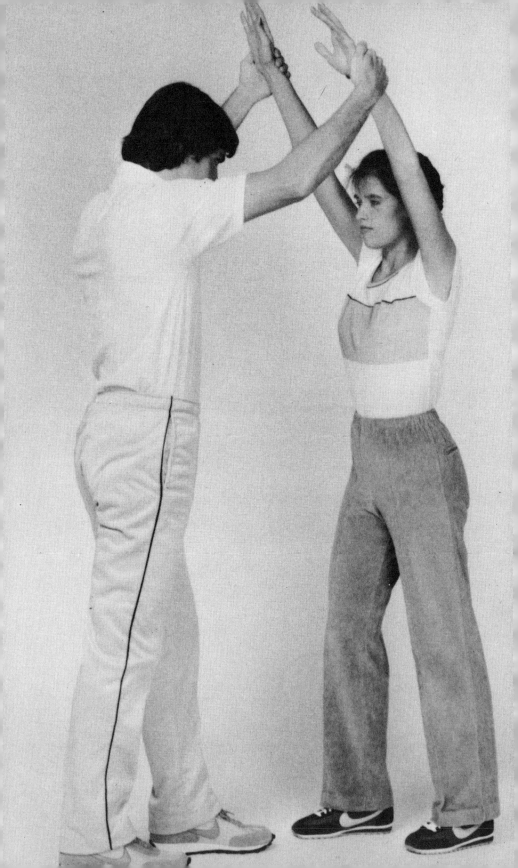

4

THE CHALLENGE

Manual resistance is an excellent alternative to the other more conventional forms of strength training methods which use costly equipment. While there are disadvantages to using MR, you should remember that there are also disadvantages to using any piece of conventional equipment. All have assets and limitations. For MR, however, the advantages far outweigh the disadvantages. MR can be performed by individuals of all ages—men and women alike. It can be done in the home, on the athletic field, or in the classroom. MR readily adapts to groups of individuals with different existing levels of fitness. No expensive equipment is necessary. MR need not replace equipment already available. It can supplement the existing equipment and serve as a productive alternative when equipment is not available. In short, it is a terrific technique for developing maximum fitness. Why not start today? The need is there. The way is clear. Manual resistance will serve you well.

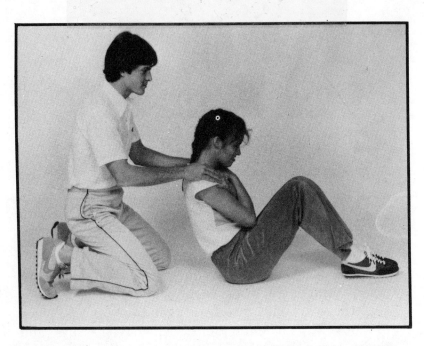

MAXIMUM MUSCULAR FITNESS:

How to Develop Strength Without Equipment